MEMORY
MEMORY
RESCUE

Questionnaires & Workbook

CONTENTS

PART I: GETTING STARTED ON YOUR MEMORY RESCUE PLAN	04
Introduction	04
Assess Where You Are Now	05
Assessment 1. Do You Have Any Early Warning Signs of Memory Problems?	05
Assessment 2. How Is Your Brain Performing?	08
Assessment 3. What Is Your Risk of Memory Problems?	10
Assessment 4. What Are Your Health "Stats"?	13
Part II: THE BRIGHT MINDS RISK FACTORS AND REMEDIES	19
Chapter 1 Risk Factor: Blood Flow	19
Chapter 2 Risk Factor: Retirement/Aging	24
Chapter 3 Risk Factor: Inflammation	28
Chapter 4 Risk Factor: Genetics	32
Chapter 5 Risk Factor: Head Trauma	35
Chapter 6 Risk Factor: Toxins	38
Chapter 7 Risk Factor: Mental Health	44
Chapter 8 Risk Factor: Immunity/Infection Issues	49
Chapter 9 Risk Factor: Neurohormone Deficiencies	52
Chapter 10 Risk Factor: Diabesity	56
Chapter 11 Risk Factor: Sleep Issues	59
PART III: 12 WEEKS TO A BETTER MEMORY	63
PART IV: RESOURCES	68

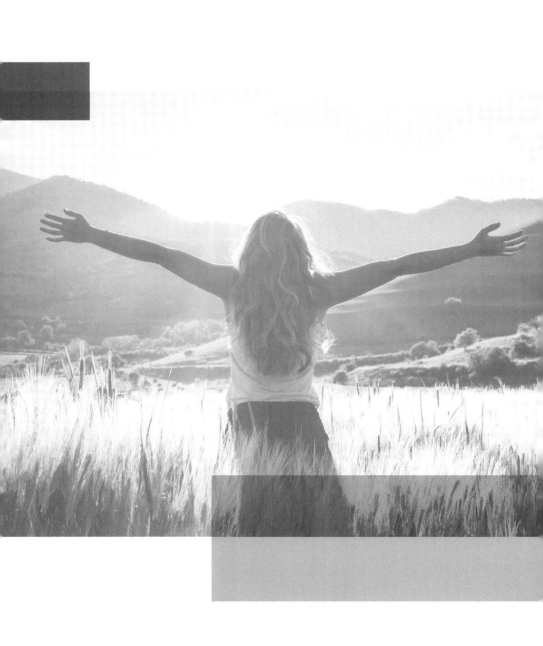

PART I:
GETTING STARTED ON YOUR MEMORY RESCUE PLAN

INTRODUCTION

How to Use This Journal to Rescue Your Memory by Supercharging Your Brain

Congratulations! You are taking a momentous step to stop memory loss, aging and Alzheimer's disease by improving the health of your brain. When your brain is working optimally, your memory works well too. You don't have trouble remembering people's names, where you put your car keys, or whether or not you turned off the stove. Although memory problems are common as you age, they are not inevitable. This journal, the companion to Memory Rescue, is designed to help you on the path to a healthier brain, a better memory and a happier, more fulfilling life.

The best way to prevent and even reverse significant memory problems is to identify them as early as possible and work to eliminate or treat all of the risk factors that may be contributing to them. The mnemonic or memory device in Memory Rescue that sums up all of these risk factors is BRIGHT MINDS.

Here are the BRIGHT MINDS risk factors that you will learn more about in this workbook and that are key to addressing memory issues:

B — Blood Flow
R — Retirement and Aging
I — Inflammation
G — Genetics
H — Head Trauma
T — Toxins

M — Mental Health
I — Immunity/Infection Issues
N — Neurohormone Deficiencies
D — Diabesity
S — Sleep Issues

Fortunately, almost all of these risk factors are either preventable or treatable, and even the ones that aren't, such as having a family history of dementia (genetics), can be improved with the right strategies. We're going to provide you with all the strategies you need to address your personal risks.

WHICH BRAIN DO YOU WANT?

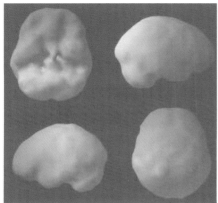 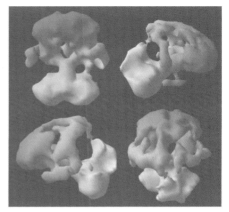

Healthy
Full, even, symmetrical blood flow

Classic Alzheimer's Disease
Decreases in parietal/temporal lobes

ASSESS WHERE YOU ARE NOW

How is your memory today? How well is your brain working? You need to answer these questions in order to determine where to devote your health-improvement efforts. That is why you will start by assessing how your brain, memory, and health are right now. Following are the assessment tools we use at Amen Clinics with all of our patients who come in with memory problems. Take the time to fill them out now (and note that you will do a reassessment in 12 weeks).

ASSESSMENT 1.
Do You Have Any Early Warning Signs of Memory Problems?

Trouble in the brain usually starts years before you have any symptoms. That's why it is so important to recognize the early warning signs. The self-assessment here includes questions relating to the most critical of these signs. (Scoring follows the questions.)

Answer each question with a number from 0-4, ranging from Never (0) to Very Frequently (4).

0	1	2	3	4
Never	Rarely	Occasionally	Frequently	Very Frequently

PROBLEMS WITH YOUR MEMORY—DO YOU:
1. _3_ Tend to be forgetful?
2. _3_ Notice that your memory, although never good, has gotten worse?
3. _1_ Misplace your keys or wallet?
4. _2_ Wonder why you came into a room?
5. _4_ Have trouble remembering names?
6. _1_ Feel embarrassed about forgetting appointments?
7. _0_ Read a book or an article, but don't remember much of it?
8. _2_ Have trouble remembering things that happened recently?
9. _1_ Struggle with brain fog?
10. _0_ Have trouble remembering to take medications or supplements?
11. _1_ Rely more and more on memory aids or reminders on your phone?
12. _1_ Know something one day but forget it the next?
13. _0_ Forget what you're going to say right in the middle of saying it?
14. _0_ Have trouble following directions that have more than one or two steps?
15. _1_ Worry that your memory is worse than it was 10 years ago?
16. _0_ Lose track of the conversation?
17. _0_ Find things in unusual places, like your keys in the refrigerator?
18. _0_ Get mad at others, thinking they took your things, only to find out later you misplaced them?

PLANNING AND PROBLEM-SOLVING ISSUES—DO YOU:
19. _0_ Have trouble making plans and sticking to them?
20. _0_ Find it harder to follow a recipe or directions on putting something together?
21. _1_ Find it hard to focus on more complex tasks, especially those that involve math? For example, are you struggling with managing your bills or balancing your checkbook?

MIX-UPS WITH TIMES AND PLACES—DO YOU:
22. _0_ Have trouble driving to locations that were once familiar to you?
23. _0_ Get easily confused or out of sorts?
24. _0_ Get more easily lost or have to rely on GPS more than before?

ISSUES WITH WORDS—DO YOU:
25. _2_ Struggle to find the right word?
26. _1_ Call things by the wrong name?
27. _0_ Avoid joining conversations with people?
28. _0_ Have trouble following along in conversations?
29. _0_ Keep repeating yourself?

JUDGMENT ISSUES—DO YOU:
30. _0_ Struggle with making more bad decisions?
31. _1_ Make mistakes with your finances?

WITHDRAWING SOCIALLY—DO YOU:
32. _0_ Feel more isolated from friends?
33. _0_ Feel like cutting back at work because you just don't care as much?
34. _0_ Feel less interested in activities you usually find fun?
35. _0_ Take less care of your physical appearance?

SCORING:
Add up the number of questions to which you answered 3 (Frequently) or 4 (Very Frequently), then check the total against the key.

KEY:
0	low risk of significant memory issues.
1-2	mild risk of having significant memory issues.
3-5	moderate risk of having significant memory issues.
6 or higher	high risk of having significant memory issues.

ASSESSMENT 2.

How Is Your Brain Performing?

Is your brain currently functioning well or not so well compared to other people your age? Cognitive testing can provide an answer. Several cognitive tests are available online; the one we use at Amen Clinics is BrainFit WebNeuro (you can access it through our BrainFitLife program at www.mybrainfitlife.com). The test takes a little more than a half hour to complete, measures an extensive number of cognitive and emotional functions, and produces an objective assessment of how your brain is working in 17 areas. Each area is scored on a scale of 1 to 10, and there is an overall brain health score as well. Any individual scores that are below 5 should raise a red flag.

The beauty of this kind of testing is that it gives you a baseline and, through repeat testing, a way to determine whether your brain is improving or deteriorating over time. (The BrainFitLife program provides specific, enjoyable brain games to strengthen any areas of weakness or vulnerability.)

Take this or another test now and repeat it in 12 weeks to chart your progress.

MY COGNITIVE TEST SCORES

My score now: _____	Motor Coordination
My score now: _____	Processing Speed (how quickly you process information)
My score now: _____	Sustained Attention (maintain focus)
My score now: _____	Controlled Attention (ability to stop reactions when needed)
My score now: _____	Flexibility (shifting attention)

My score now:_____	Inhibition (self-control)
My score now:_____	Working Memory (hold information for short periods)
My score now:_____	Recall Memory (remember information)
My score now:_____	Executive Function (plan and organize information
My score now:_____	Identify Emotions (reading faces)
My score now:_____	Emotion Bias (impact of emotions on decision making)
My score now:_____	Stress Level
My score now:_____	Anxiety Level
My score now:_____	Depressed Mood Level
My score now:_____	Positivity-Negativity Bias (tendency to notice positive or negative emotions)
My score now:_____	Resilience (coping during times of trial)
My score now:_____	Social Capacity (building and keeping relationships)
My score now:_____	**OVERALL BRAIN HEALTH**

ASSESSMENT 3.
What Is Your Risk of Alzheimer's Disease and Memory Problems?

Alzheimer's disease (AD) is the most common type of dementia, affecting more than 5 million people in the U.S.—a number expected to triple by the year 2050. It is the third leading cause of death, and there is currently no cure.

Research has confirmed that the best way to prevent AD and memory loss is to prevent all the illnesses that put you at risk for it. Therefore, if you want to keep your brain healthy as you get older, it is critical to avoid the risk factors as much as possible.

Here are the key risk factors, according to the BRIGHT MINDS formula. Each contributing factor has been given a numerical weighting that indicates how harmful it may be to your brain and memory. Check off the contributing risks that you know apply to you. If you don't know if you have a risk factor (which may rely upon the results of certain lab tests), consult the appropriate Memory Rescue chapter for further information. When you have finished this questionnaire, go back and tally your score. The number in the right column is the relative increase in risk for memory troubles, accelerated aging, and Alzheimer's compared to people who don't have that risk factor.

This is what the numbers mean:
1.3 = 30% increased risk
1.7 = 70% increased risk
2 = twice the risk
4 = quadruple the risk, and on up to 38 = 38 times the risk!

BLOOD FLOW RISK FACTORS
- ☐ History of a stroke — 5
- ☐ History of cardiovascular disease, including coronary artery disease, heart attacks, heart failure, heart arrhythmias — 2
- ☐ Prehypertension or hypertension in midlife — 2
- ☐ Low blood pressure in later life — 1.3

- ☐ Erectile dysfunction
  - •All ages   1.7
  - •Age 50 to 64   6.1
  - •Over age 65   27.2
- ☐ Limited exercise (under 2 times a week)   2

RETIREMENT/AGING RISK FACTORS

- ☐ Age 65 to 84   2
- ☐ Age 85 and older   38
- ☐ Watching too much television (more than 2 hours a day)   2
- ☐ A job that does not require new learning, or retired without new opportunities for learning   2
- ☐ Loneliness or social isolation   2

INFLAMMATION RISK FACTORS

- ☐ Periodontal (gum) disease   2
- ☐ Presence of inflammation in the body, such as high homocysteine or C-reactive protein   2
- ☐ Low omega-3 fatty acids (from Omega-3 Index test)   2

GENETICS RISK FACTORS

- ☐ One family member with Alzheimer's or dementia   3.5
- ☐ More than one family member with Alzheimer's or dementia   7.5
- ☐ One apolipoprotein E (APOE) e4 gene (if known, based on genetic testing)   2.5
- ☐ Two APOE e4 genes (if known, based on genetic testing)   10

HEAD TRAUMA RISK FACTORS

- ☐ A single head injury with loss of consciousness   2
- ☐ Several head injuries without a loss of consciousness   2
- ☐ Loss of one's sense of smell   2

TOXIN RISK FACTORS

- ☐ Smoking cigarettes for 10 years or longer (currently or in past)   2.3
- ☐ Alcohol dependence or drug dependence (currently or in past)   4.4
- ☐ History of radiation for head and neck cancers   3
- ☐ History of chemotherapy
  - •For breast cancer   1.5
  - •For colorectal cancer, possibly other cancers   1.25

- ☐ Chronic exposure to heavy metals, such as lead, cadmium, mercury, arsenic, or aluminum — 1.5
- ☐ Chronic mold exposure — 1.5
- ☐ Kidney dysfunction — 2

MENTAL HEALTH RISK FACTORS

- ☐ PTSD — 4
- ☐ Bipolar disorder — 2
- ☐ Schizophrenia — 2
- ☐ Depression — 3.5
- ☐ Chronic stress — 2

IMMUNITY/INFECTION ISSUES

- ☐ Autoimmune issues, including
  - Multiple sclerosis — 1.5
  - Rheumatoid arthritis — 3
  - Systemic lupus erythematosus — 2
  - Crohn's disease — 1.5
  - Severe psoriasis — 3
- ☐ Adult asthma — 1.3
- ☐ Chronic Lyme disease or other infectious process in brain/body not fully treated — 2
- ☐ Cold sores or genital herpes — 2

NEUROHORMONE RISK FACTORS

- ☐ Low in thyroid — 2
- ☐ Low estrogen (in females) — 2
- ☐ Low testosterone (males and females) — 2
- ☐ Hysterectomy without estrogen replacement — 2
- ☐ History of prostate cancer with testosterone-lowering treatment — 2

DIABESITY RISK FACTORS

- ☐ Pre-diabetes or diabetes — 3
- ☐ Being overweight or obese in middle age — 3
- ☐ Being underweight in older age — 2

SLEEP RISK FACTORS

- ☐ Chronic insomnia — 2.3
- ☐ Sleep apnea — 2

TOTAL YOUR SCORE:

Tally the number of risk factors you have checked off and then tally the numbers for the risk factors you checked (relative risk factors).

___ **Total number of risk factors (number of checked boxes)**

___ **Relative risk factors (total from the relevant numbers in the right-hand column)**

HOW TO INTERPRET YOUR RELATIVE RISK FACTOR SCORE

0-6 You likely have a low risk of developing AD.

7-14 You have a moderate risk; consider annual screening* after age 50.

14+ Consider annual screening* after age 40.

*Annual screening should include lab tests, a repeat of cognitive testing and a checkup with your healthcare provider.

ASSESSMENT 4.
What Are Your Health "Stats"?

These numbers let you know how your body is functioning and are common yet important indicators of your overall health. In the chart that follows, enter the numbers that you know or can assess yourself; for those that you don't know, you will need to have your blood drawn (ask your doctor to order this for you or visit one of the Amen Clinics). Enter these numbers in the chart when you receive your test results.

MY IMPORTANT HEALTH NUMBERS

Let's start with your Body Mass Index (BMI). Find your height in the left column, and then read across that row to find your weight. Your BMI is at the top of that column.

Obese (>30)   Overweight (>25-30)   Normal (>18.5-25)   Underweight (<18.5)

WEIGHT   **HEIGHT** in feet, inches and centimeters

lbs	4'8" 142cm	4'9" 149	4'10" 147	4'11" 150	5'0" 152	5'1" 155	5'2" 157	5'3" 160	5'4" 163	5'5" 165	5'6" 168	5'7" 170	5'8" 173	5'9" 175	5'10" 178	5'11" 180	6'0" 183	6'1" 185	6'2" 188	6'3" 191	6'4" 193	6'5" 196
260	58	56	54	53	51	49	48	46	45	43	42	41	40	38	37	36	35	34	33	32	32	31
255	57	55	53	51	50	48	47	45	44	42	41	40	39	38	37	36	35	34	33	32	31	30
250	56	54	52	50	49	47	46	44	43	42	40	39	38	37	36	35	34	33	32	31	30	30
245	55	53	51	49	48	46	45	43	42	41	40	38	37	36	35	34	33	32	31	31	30	29
240	54	52	50	48	47	45	44	43	41	40	39	38	36	35	34	33	33	32	31	30	29	28
235	53	51	49	47	46	44	43	42	40	39	38	37	36	35	34	33	32	31	30	29	29	28
230	52	50	48	46	45	43	42	41	39	38	37	36	35	34	33	32	31	30	30	29	28	27
225	50	49	47	45	44	43	41	40	39	37	36	35	34	33	32	31	31	30	29	28	27	27
220	49	48	46	44	43	42	40	39	38	37	36	34	33	32	32	31	30	29	28	27	27	26
215	48	47	45	43	42	41	39	38	37	36	35	34	33	32	31	30	29	28	28	27	26	25
210	47	45	44	42	41	40	38	37	36	35	34	33	32	31	30	29	28	28	27	26	26	25
205	46	44	43	41	40	39	37	36	35	34	33	32	31	30	29	29	28	27	26	26	25	24
200	45	43	42	40	39	38	37	35	34	33	32	31	30	30	29	28	27	26	26	25	24	24
195	44	42	41	39	38	37	36	35	33	32	31	31	30	29	28	27	26	26	25	24	24	23
190	43	41	40	38	37	36	35	34	33	32	31	30	29	28	27	26	26	25	24	24	23	23
185	41	40	39	37	36	35	34	33	32	31	30	29	28	27	27	26	25	24	24	23	23	22
180	40	39	38	36	35	34	33	32	31	30	29	28	27	27	26	25	24	24	23	22	22	21
175	39	38	37	35	34	33	32	31	30	29	28	27	27	26	25	24	24	23	22	22	21	21
170	38	37	36	34	33	32	31	30	29	28	27	27	26	25	24	24	23	22	22	21	21	20
165	37	36	34	33	32	31	30	29	28	27	27	26	25	24	24	23	22	22	21	21	20	20
160	36	35	33	32	31	30	29	28	27	27	26	25	24	24	23	22	22	21	21	20	19	19
155	35	34	32	31	30	29	28	27	27	26	25	24	24	23	22	22	21	20	20	19	19	18
150	34	32	31	30	29	28	27	27	26	25	24	23	23	22	22	21	20	20	19	19	18	18
145	33	31	30	29	28	27	27	26	25	24	23	23	22	21	21	20	20	19	19	18	18	17
140	31	30	29	28	27	26	26	25	24	23	23	22	21	21	20	20	19	18	18	17	17	17
135	30	29	28	27	26	26	25	24	23	22	22	21	21	20	19	19	18	18	17	17	16	16
130	29	28	27	26	25	25	24	23	22	22	21	20	20	19	19	18	18	17	17	16	16	15
125	28	27	26	25	24	24	23	22	21	21	20	20	19	18	18	17	17	16	16	16	15	15
120	27	26	25	24	23	23	22	21	21	20	19	19	18	18	17	17	16	16	15	15	15	14
115	26	25	24	23	22	22	21	20	20	19	19	18	17	17	16	16	16	15	15	14	14	14
110	25	24	23	22	21	21	20	19	19	18	18	17	17	16	16	15	15	15	14	14	13	13
105	24	23	22	21	21	20	19	19	18	17	17	16	16	16	15	15	14	14	13	13	13	12
100	22	22	21	20	20	19	18	18	17	17	16	16	15	15	14	14	14	13	13	12	12	12
95	21	21	20	19	19	18	17	17	16	16	15	15	14	14	14	13	13	13	12	12	12	11
90	20	19	19	18	18	17	16	16	15	15	15	14	14	13	13	13	12	12	12	11	11	11
85	19	18	18	17	17	16	16	15	15	14	14	13	13	13	12	12	12	11	11	11	10	10
80	18	17	17	16	16	15	15	14	14	13	13	13	12	12	11	11	11	11	10	10	10	9

My Body Mass Index Number: _____	**BODY MASS INDEX (BMI):** Underweight: Under 19 Normal weight: 19-24.9 Overweight: 25-29.9 Obese: 30 or higher Morbid obesity: 40 or higher
My WTHR Number: _____	**WAIST TO HEIGHT RATIO (WTHR):** Use a tape measure to measure at your belly button. For a healthy WtHR, your waist size should be half your height—or less—in inches **HEALTHY RATIO:** Less than or equal to 0.5.
My Blood Pressure Number: _____	**BLOOD PRESSURE:** **OPTIMAL** Systolic (top number): 90-120 Diastolic (bottom number): 60-80

My Cholesterol Number:
_____
	LIPID PANEL (CHOLESTEROL):
	- Total cholesterol:
	  Normal: 135-200 mg/dL (below 135 has been associated with depression)
	  Optimal: 160-200 mg/dL
	- **HDL:** greater than or equal to 60 mg/dL
	- **LDL:** less than 100 mg/dL
	- Triglycerides: less than 150 mg/dl

My General Metabolic Numbers:	**GENERAL METABOLIC PANEL (KIDNEY AND LIVER FUNCTION):**
ALT (SGPT) _____ **AST (SGOT)** _____ **Bilirubin** _____ **Zinc** _____ **BUN**_____ **Creatinine**_____	LIVER FUNCTION ☐ **ALT (SGPT):** Normal range: 7 to 56 units per liter (U/L) ☐ **AST (SGOT):** Normal range: 5 to 40 U/L ☐ **Bilirubin:** Normal range: 0.2 to 1.2 mg/dL ☐ **Zinc:** Normal range: 60 to 110 mcg/dL (low zinc will limit detoxification in the liver) KIDNEY FUNCTION ☐ **BUN:** Normal range: 7 to 20 mg/dL ☐ **Creatinine:** Normal range: 0.5 to 1.2 mg/dL
My Fasting Blood Sugar Number: _____	**FASTING BLOOD SUGAR:** **Normal:** 70-105 mg/dL **Optimal:** 70-85 mg/dL **Pre-diabetes:** 105-125 mg/dL **Diabetes:** 126 mg/dL or higher
My HbA1c Number: _____	**HEMOGLOBIN A1C (HBA1C):** **Normal:** 4.0 – 5.6% **Prediabetes:** 5.7 – 6.4%
My Homocysteine Number: _____	**HOMOCYSTEINE:** **Healthy level:** less than 10 mmol/L

My C-Reactive Protein Number: _____	**C-REACTIVE PROTEIN:** Healthy range: 0.0 - 1.0 mg/dL
My Ferritin Number: _____	**FERRITIN:** Ideal levels: 40–80 ng/mL
My Thyroid Numbers: TSH:_____ Free T3:_____ Free T4:_____	**THYROID:** Thyroid-stimulating hormone (TSH): 0.4–3.0mIU/L Free T3: 100–200ng/dL Free T4: 4.5–11.2mcg/dL
My Free Serum Testosterone Number: _____ **My Total Serum Testosterone Number:**_____	**FREE & TOTAL SERUM TESTOSTERONE:** Normal levels for women: Free: 0.3-1.9 ng/dL Total: 8-60 ng/dL Optimal levels for women: Free:0.8-1.9ng/dL Total:30-60ng/dL Normal levels for men: Free: 9-30 ng/dL Total: 300-1100 ng/dL Optimal levels for men: Free: 15-30 ng/dL Total: 600-1100 ng/dL
My DHEA-S Number: _____	**DHEA-S:** Normal: 44–332 µg/dL
My Vitamin D Number: _____	**VITAMIN D:** Low: Below 30mg/dL Optimal: 50-100mg/dL

SELF-ASSESSMENT RECAP

1. Note any signs of memory loss that you are experiencing.
2. Take an online cognitive test to see how your brain is functioning compared to others your age.
3. Find out what your personal BRIGHT MINDS risk factors and relative risks are.
4. Know your important health numbers and record them.

MEET SAM AND SCARLETT, THE SEAHORSE TWINS

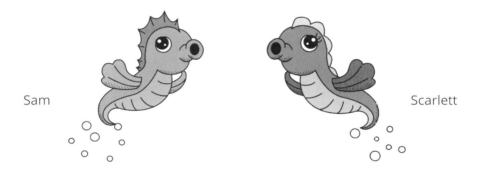

Sam   Scarlett

You first met Sam and Scarlett in chapter 20 of Memory Rescue. They embody a significant brain structure called the hippocampus—the Latin word for seahorse. You have two of these structures (or "hippocampi"), one within each of the temporal lobes. They are critical in the processing of memories and in your responses to emotional stimuli. Because of their important role in the health of your brain, Scarlett and Sam will provide tips and insights to help you make the most of this workbook.

PART II:
THE BRIGHT MINDS RISK FACTORS AND REMEDIES

CHAPTER 1

RISK FACTOR: BLOOD FLOW

Blood flow throughout your body brings oxygen and other nutrients to all your cells and carries away waste products. Surprisingly, the blood vessels that feed our brain cells age faster than those neurons, so keeping your brain healthy means taking care of your blood vessels.

YOUR PERSONAL RISK CHECKLIST:
Which Blood Flow Risk Factors Do You Have?

If you are unsure whether you have any of the following risk factors, schedule a checkup with your healthcare provider, who will take your blood pressure, listen to your heart and order laboratory tests to assess the health of your blood vessels. You can always fill in this checklist when you have the results of your checkup and tests.

CARDIOVASCULAR DISEASE
- ☐ Atherosclerosis (hardening of the arteries)
- ☐ High LDL or total cholesterol
- ☐ Heart attack
- ☐ Atrial fibrillation
- ☐ Hypertension or prehypertension
    - •Hypertensive: 140/90 mm/mg or higher
    - •Prehypertensive: 80/120 – 89/139 mm/mg

OTHER RISK FACTORS
- ☐ Having a stroke or transient ischemic attack (TIA)
- ☐ Exercising less than twice a week and/or a slow walking speed. Ultimately, one of the most important reasons to exercise is that it keeps your blood vessels open and healthy.
- ☐ Erectile dysfunction
- ☐ Episode(s) of a loss of oxygen to the brain (such as during sleep apnea, a near drowning or a heart attack, when the heart stops beating)

KEY BLOOD FLOW TESTS

While it is important to know all of your health numbers, the ones here are key to assessing the status of your circulatory system. Be sure to have these tests done now.

- ☐ Blood pressure: Both high and low blood pressure (less than 90/60) are a problem
- ☐ CBC (complete blood count)
- ☐ Lipid panel: Cholesterol levels that are too high or too low are bad for the brain

HOW TO ADDRESS YOUR RISKS

THE RISK:	Stroke, heart disease, atrial fibrillation, high cholesterol, prehypertension or hypertension, erectile dysfunction
THE RESCUE:	<ul><li>Get treatment and start prevention strategies early.</li><li>Lose weight if you are overweight (BMI over 25)</li><li>Eat a nutrient-rich diet that tames inflammation</li><li>Get 7-8 hours of sleep every night</li><li>Meditate or pray for 10-20 minutes daily</li></ul>
THE RISK:	Exercising less than twice a week or for less than 30 minutes a session.

THE RESCUE:	<ul><li>Burst or Interval Training: Alternate 1-minute bursts of high-intensity exercise with several minutes of restful activity (e.g., do 4-5 high-speed bursts over the course of a 30-minute stationary bike ride)</li><li>Strength Training: Two 30- to 45-minute weightlifting sessions a week</li><li>Coordination Activities, such as dancing, tennis, or table tennis</li><li>Mindful Exercise, such as yoga and Tai Chi</li></ul>
THE RISK:	Drinking too much caffeine, sugar-sweetened and diet sodas, and/or alcohol; eating baked goods, fast foods, fried foods, and trans fats
THE RESCUE:	<ul><li>Avoid or eliminate alcohol, caffeine, fruit juices, and sodas (including diet sodas)</li><li>Drink plenty of water</li><li>Avoid or eliminate baked goods, fast foods, fried foods, and trans fats</li><li>Limit salt intake to 1,500-2,300 mg. a day</li><li>Eat more plant-based foods for their fiber and healthy nutrients, which improve blood flow</li><li>Consider blood pressure-lowering supplements: magnesium, potassium, CoQ10, vitamins C and D, and aged garlic</li></ul>
THE RISK:	Sleep apnea or other loss of oxygen
THE RESCUE:	Consider hyperbaric oxygen therapy (HBOT)

CAPITALIZE ON THE BLOOD FLOW BENEFITS OF EXERCISE

Here are just a few of the ways in which exercise can help your blood vessels and your brain.

- It improves blood pressure
- It improves the heart's ability to pump blood throughout the body and brain, which increases oxygen and nutrient delivery
- It boosts the flexibility of blood vessels, which decreases the risk for high blood pressure, stroke and heart disease
- It stimulates the brain's ability to grow new brain cells, or neurons
- It improves mood, focus and cognitive flexibility

SCARLETT SAYS: *Get moving! Exercise helps boost the size of your hippocampus. For women, even a leisurely walk has benefits.*

CONSIDER TAKING NUTRACEUTICALS THAT IMPROVE BLOOD FLOW

- ✓ Ginkgo biloba extract: 60 to 120 mg twice a day
- ✓ Cocoa flavanols: 1 oz. of sugar-free, dairy-free dark chocolate every day
- ✓ Omega-3 fatty acids: 1,400 mg (or more) per day in roughly a 60/40 EPA:DHA ratio
- ✓ Green tea catechins (GTC): Up to 600 mg a day
- ✓ Resveratrol: 75 mg a day
- ✓ Probiotics: 3 billion live organisms a day, with both Lactobacillus and Bifidobacterium bacterial strains

EAT MORE OF THESE HEART-HEALTHY FOODS AND SPICES

Arginine-rich foods: beets (and beet juice), pork, turkey, chicken, beef, salmon, halibut, trout, steel-cut oats, clams, watermelon, pistachios, walnuts, seeds, kale, spinach, celery, cabbage, and radishes

Foods rich in vitamin B6, B12, and folate: leafy greens, cabbage, bok choy, bell peppers, cauliflower, lentils, asparagus, garbanzo beans, spinach, broccoli, parsley, cauliflower, salmon, sardines, lamb, tuna, beef, and eggs

Vitamin E–rich foods: green leafy vegetables, almonds, hazelnuts, and sunflower seeds

Magnesium-rich foods: pumpkin and sunflower seeds, almonds, spinach, Swiss chard, sesame seeds, beet greens, summer squash, quinoa, black beans, and cashews

Potassium-rich foods: beet greens, Swiss chard, spinach, bok choy, beets, Brussels sprouts, broccoli, celery, cantaloupe, tomatoes, salmon, banana, onions, green peas, sweet potato, avocados, and lentils

Fiber: see chapter 10

Garlic

Vitamin C–rich foods: see chapter 8

Polyphenol-rich foods: see chapter 4

Omega 3–rich foods: see chapter 3

Maca: a root vegetable native to Peru

Spices: cayenne pepper, ginger, garlic, turmeric, coriander and cardamom, cinnamon, rosemary, and bergamot

CHAPTER 2

RISK FACTOR: RETIREMENT AND AGING

Advancing age is the single most important risk for memory loss and Alzheimer's disease. While that is true, it's not inevitable that your mental faculties decline with age. Keeping mentally fit means addressing the biological and emotional/psychological issues that arise as you get older.

YOUR PERSONAL RISK CHECKLIST: WHICH RETIREMENT/AGING RISK FACTORS DO YOU HAVE?

If you are unsure whether you have any of the following risk factors, schedule a checkup with your healthcare provider, who can order laboratory tests for iron and other health measures related to aging. You can always fill in this checklist when you have the results of your checkup and tests.

- ☐ Age: I am ___ years old
- ☐ Retirement/lack of new learning
- ☐ Social isolation
- ☐ Too much (or too little) iron
- ☐ Shortened telomeres (casings at the ends of chromosomes)

KEY RETIREMENT/AGING TESTS

While it is important to know all of your health numbers, the ones here are key to assessing how well you are aging. Be sure to have these tests done now.

- ☐ C-reactive protein (CRP): a measure of inflammation
- ☐ Fasting blood sugar: This blood test, along with Hemoglobin A1c, screens for prediabetes and diabetes
- ☐ Hemoglobin A1C (HbA1C)
- ☐ DHEA: Higher levels of this neurohormone, as well as testosterone, are associated with longevity
- ☐ Testosterone
- ☐ Ferritin (iron levels)
- ☐ Telomere length: Testing for CRP and HbA1C (see above) may be substituted for this test

SAM SAYS: *Be careful not to use "old people's speech." Saying you're too old or too tired or too set in your ways can be a self-fulfilling prophecy!*

HOW TO ADDRESS YOUR RISKS

THE RISK:	Retirement, social isolation and loneliness
THE RESCUE:	☐ Get involved with your family, church, or other groups ☐ Take a class (to meet other and engage in new learning) ☐ Get physically active ☐ Form new friendships ☐ Volunteer to help others
THE RISK:	Too much (or too little) iron
THE RESCUE:	If your iron level is too high: • Limit alcohol consumption (it increases absorption of iron from your diet) • Check your multivitamin/mineral to see if it's high in iron • Limit cooking in iron pans • Read labels of foods like cereal to see if they are "iron fortified" and avoid them if they are

THE RESCUE:	- Avoid foods with naturally high levels of iron: red meat, spinach, chard, cumin, lentils, chickpeas, broccoli, soybeans, collard greens, leeks, beans, sprouts, asparagus, kelp, pumpkin and sesame seeds, and olives - Consider donating blood If your iron level is too low: - Consider taking an iron supplement
THE RISK:	Shrinking telomeres (casings at the ends of chromosomes)
THE RESCUE:	- Avoid sodas, trans fats, processed foods, alcohol - Lose weight if you are overweight - Get 7 to 8 hours of sleep a night - Give up cigarette smoking - Treat infections promptly - Avoid exposure to heavy metals - Eat plenty of antioxidant-rich foods and spices - Exercise - Address your stress: learn stress reduction techniques and/or mindfulness meditation - Take a multivitamin/mineral daily

CONSIDER TAKING NUTRACEUTICALS THAT HELP IMPROVE YOUR MEMORY AND BRAIN FUNCTION

- ✓ **Alpha GPC (alpha-glycerylphosphorylcholine):** 600 mg once or twice a day
- ✓ **Phosphatidylserine (PS):** 200 to 300 mg a day
- ✓ **Acetyl-L-carnitine (ALCAR):** 500 to 2,000 mg a day
- ✓ **N-acetylcysteine (NAC):** 600 to 1,800 mg a day; try starting at 600 mg twice a day
- ✓ **Huperzine A:** 50 to 100 mcg twice a day
- ✓ **Saffron:** 30 mg a day of a concentrate produced from the flower; 176.5 mg a day of Satiereal (patented preparation)
- ✓ **Bacopa (bacopa monnieri):** 250 to 500 mg per day of the standardized extract Synapsa
- ✓ **Sage:** 300 to 600 mg of dried sage leaf in capsules, or 25 to 50 microliters (mcL); use only under a physician's supervision if you have high blood pressure or a seizure disorder

SCARLETT SAYS: *Try fasting for 12 to 16 hours a night to help your brain clean up its toxic trash. If you eat dinner at 7 p.m., plan to have breakfast sometime between 7 and 11 a.m.*

EAT MORE OF THESE ANTI-AGING FOODS AND SPICES

Antioxidant-rich spices: cloves, oregano, rosemary, thyme, cinnamon, turmeric, sage, garlic, ginger, fennel

Antioxidant-rich foods: acai fruit, parsley, cocoa powder, raspberries, walnuts, blueberries, artichokes, cranberries, kidney beans, blackberries, pomegranates, chocolate, olive and hemp oil (don't use either oil for cooking at high temperatures), dandelion greens, green tea

Choline-rich foods: to support acetylcholine and memory: shrimp, eggs, scallops, chicken, turkey, beef, cod, salmon, shiitake mushrooms, chickpeas, lentils, collard greens

Allicin-rich foods: See chapter 9.

Polyphenols-rich foods: See chapter 5.

Foods rich in vitamin B12 and folate: See chapter 2.

CHAPTER 3

RISK FACTOR: INFLAMMATION

The root of the word inflammation is the Latin inflammare, which means "to set on fire." That describes what chronic inflammation does inside your body. It is like a constant fire that harms your organs and can destroy your brain.

YOUR PERSONAL RISK CHECKLIST:
Which Inflammation Risk Factors Do You Have?

While inflammation is your body's natural (and necessary) reaction to infection and injury, it's important to know what else can trigger inflammation and the conditions under which it can become chronic and harmful. Cigarette smoking, high blood sugar levels, exposure to environmental toxins, and gum disease are a few of the culprits. The following are two major memory-harming sources of chronic inflammation:

- ☐ Leaky gut (when the lining of the gastrointestinal tract becomes permeable)
- ☐ Low omega-3 fatty acids (especially the fatty acids known as EPA and DHA)

SCARLETT SAYS: *Your friendly gut bacteria can help you fight off illness-causing bacterial like E. coli and fend off anxious, stressed, tired, or depressed feelings.*

KEY TESTS FOR INFLAMMATION

While it is important to know all of your health numbers, the ones here are key to assessing whether or not inflammation is an issue for you. Be sure to have these blood tests done now.

- ☐ C-reactive protein (CRP)
- ☐ Interleukin 6 (IL-6)
- ☐ Homocysteine
- ☐ Folate
- ☐ Vitamin B12
- ☐ Omega-3 Index: a measure of omega-3 fatty acids EPA and DHA in red blood cells, which reflects brain levels of these fats

HOW TO ADDRESS YOUR RISKS

THE RISK:	Leaky gut
THE RESCUE:	<ul><li>Avoid things that hurt your gut, such as medications (e.g., antibiotics, NSAIDS, proton pump inhibitors), toxins, stress, intestinal infections, gluten, excessive alcohol, and more</li><li>Increase the healthy bacteria in your gastrointestinal tract by taking a probiotic supplement or eating fermented foods with live bacteria (kefir, kombucha, pickled fruits/veggies, unsweetened yogurt)</li><li>Eat more prebiotics, such as beans, apples, onions, and root veggies, which feed good probiotic bacteria</li><li>Take antibiotics only when indicated and necessary</li></ul>

THE RISK:	Elevated homocysteine (associated with inflammation, atherosclerosis, higher risk of heart attack, stroke, blood clots, and possibly Alzheimer's disease)
THE RESCUE:	Optimize your levels of B vitamins—especially B6, B12, and folate—to help lower homocysteine
THE RISK:	Low levels of omega-3 fatty acids EPA and DHA
THE RESCUE:	<ul><li>Take a fish oil supplement that provides at least 1,000 mg of EPA plus DHA a day</li><li>Eat more cold-water fish, including salmon, tuna, mackerel, sardines, and herring. Check Seafood Watch to make sure the fish you buy isn't contaminated with mercury or other toxins</li></ul>
THE RISK:	Bleeding gums and gum disease
THE RESCUE:	<ul><li>Brush your teeth twice a day after meals and floss daily</li><li>See a dentist regularly for checkups and cleanings</li></ul>

SAM SAYS: *Aim for an Omega-3 Index of at least 8. It will keep your brain sharp and strengthen your memory.*

CONSIDER TAKING NUTRACEUTICALS

- ✓ If your homocysteine level is high, take: folate (800 micrograms [mcg] a day of methyl folate), vitamin B12 (500 mcg a day of methyl cobalamin), and vitamin B6 (20 mg a day or pyridoxine hydrochloride or pyridoxal-5-phosphate
- ✓ Omega-3 fatty acids: 1,400 to 2,800 mg a day in roughly a 60/40 EPA:DHA ratio
- ✓ Curcumin: 500 to 2,000 mg a day of a highly bioavailable supplement such as Longvida
- ✓ Probiotics: 3 billion live organisms a day; look for both Lactobacillus and Bifidobacterium bacterial strains

EAT MORE OF THESE NFLAMMATION-FIGHTING FOODS AND SPICES

Anti-inflammatory spices: turmeric, cayenne, ginger, cloves, cinnamon, oregano, pumpkin pie spice, rosemary, sage, fennel

Folate-rich foods: spinach, dark leafy greens, asparagus, turnips, beets, mustard greens, brussels sprouts, lima beans, beef liver, root vegetables, kidney beans, white beans, salmon, avocado

Omega-3-rich foods: flaxseeds, walnuts, salmon, sardines, beef, shrimp, walnut oil, chia seeds, and avocado oil. (Animal sources provide EPA and DHA directly, but plant sources have to be converted, and some people's enzyme systems are poor at making this conversion.)

Prebiotic-rich foods: dandelion greens, asparagus, chia seeds, beans, cabbage, psyllium, artichokes, raw garlic, onions, leeks, root vegetables (sweet potatoes, yams, squash, jicama, beets, carrots, turnips)

Probiotic-rich foods: brined vegetables (not vinegar), kimchi, sauerkraut, kefir, miso soup, pickles, spirulina, chlorella, blue-green algae, kombucha

Tart cherry juice: to lower CRP.

Magnesium-rich foods: See chapter 2.

Polyphenol-rich foods: See chapter 5.

Allicin-rich foods: See chapter 9.

Fiber-rich foods: See chapter 11.

CHAPTER 4

RISK FACTOR: GENETICS

Every human being inherits two sets of 23 chromosomes—one set from each parent. Genes on these chromosomes contain the instructions to produce the proteins that our cells are made of. Having a problem with your chromosomes or genes can result in health issues.

YOUR PERSONAL RISK CHECKLIST:
Which Genetic Risk Factors Do You Have?

In families that have severe memory problems, Alzheimer's disease, or dementia, members are more at risk of memory troubles. The same is true for people who have one or two copies of the APOE e4 gene or several other genes. It is therefore critical to know if your extended family members have problems with their memories and take steps to protect yours.

- ☐ A family history of memory problems, dementia, or Alzheimer's
- ☐ One or two APOE e4 genes
- ☐ Presinilin 1 or 2 genes

KEY GENETIC TESTS

- ☐ Apolipoprotein E gene (APOE) status
- ☐ Additional genetic testing (for other genes like presinilin genes 1 and 2 if members of your family have early-onset memory problems; ask your doctor about this)

HOW TO ADDRESS YOUR RISKS

THE RISK:	Family history of memory problems, dementia, or Alzheimer's disease; one or two APOE e4 genes
THE RESCUE:	<ul><li>Get screened early (around age 40) with cognitive testing, questionnaires, and even SPECT imaging</li><li>Be serious about the health of your brain: Engage in sports or hobbies that call for new learning and protect your blood vessels</li><li>Exercise aerobically, do balance exercises, and strengthen your muscles</li><li>Protect your head from injury and concussions</li></ul>

SAM SAYS: *Just because you have the APOE e4 gene doesn't mean you will develop Alzheimer's—75 percent of people who inherit the gene don't get AD. But it does mean you have to take very good care of your brain and blood vessels.*

CONSIDER TAKING NUTRACEUTICALS DAILY

- ✓ Blueberry extract
- ✓ Resveratrol
- ✓ Green tea catechins (GTC)
- ✓ Acetyl-L-carnitine (ALCAR)
- ✓ Curcumin
- ✓ Ashwagandha
- ✓ Ginseng

- ✓ N-acetylcysteine
- ✓ Coenzyme Q10 (CoQ10)
- ✓ Magnesium
- ✓ Vitamins B6 and B12
- ✓ Vitamin D
- ✓ DHA

SCARLETT SAYS: *Just say no to processed cheese and microwave popcorn! They both contain diacetyl, a flavoring that increases beta amyloid, the sticky brain substance linked to Alzheimer's.*

EAT MORE OF THESE BRAIN-BOOSTING FOODS AND SPICES

Spices to help decrease beta amyloid: sage, turmeric, cinnamon, cardamom, ginger, saffron, cinnamon (which decreases tau aggregation)

Foods to decrease beta amyloid: salmon, blueberries, curry

Polyphenol-rich foods: chocolate, green tea, blueberries, kale, red wine, onions, apples, cherries, cabbage

Vitamin B6, vitamin B12, and folate-rich foods: See chapter 2.

Magnesium-rich foods: See chapter 3

Vitamin D–rich foods: See chapter 9

A ketogenic (very low carbohydrate) diet: Shown to decrease beta amyloid in animal models

CHAPTER 5

RISK FACTOR: HEAD TRAUMA

Numerous studies have shown that a head injury—or multiple head injuries—are linked to a higher risk of memory problems. Those that occur early in life (before age 25) more than double the risk; those that happen later (after age 55) almost quadruple the risk.

YOUR PERSONAL RISK CHECKLIST:
Which Head Trauma Risk Factors Do You Have?

Brain tissue is soft, like custard, and the bony skull that protects the brain has sharp ridges. As a result, anything that causes your brain to hit up against your skull can cause trauma—bruising, bleeding, lack of oxygen, damaged brain cells, and more. Here are a few of the things that can lead to this kind of trauma:

- ☐ A fall (down steps, off a ladder, out of bed, in the bath or shower, out of a tree, etc.)
- ☐ A motor vehicle collision (with a car, motorcycle, truck, bicycle, ATV)
- ☐ A pedestrian-vehicle collision
- ☐ Sport injuries and concussions (in football, soccer, boxing, baseball, basketball, cycling, etc.)
- ☐ Combat injuries (including explosive blasts)
- ☐ Violence (gunshot wounds, domestic violence, an assault, etc.)

SAM SAYS: *If you have kids who want to play football, first explain why it's a bad idea if they want to grow up to be healthy and happy. Then tell them "no."*

KEY TESTS FOR HEAD TRAUMA

- ☐ If you have had a head trauma and your memory isn't what you want it to be or if your thinking skills are impaired, consider getting a SPECT or QEEG scan
- ☐ Check out your sense of smell if you are having trouble smelling peanut butter, lemon, strawberry or natural gas scents
- ☐ Omega-3 Index
- ☐ HbA1c and fasting blood sugar (high blood sugar levels can delay healing)
- ☐ Thyroid, DHEA, and testosterone levels (damage to the master hormone gland, the pituitary, can cause hormone deficiencies)

HOW TO ADDRESS YOUR RISKS

THE RISK:	Sustaining an injury to your head
THE RESCUE:	<ul><li>Refrain from playing contact sports</li><li>Use a helmet when you go skiing, biking, etc.</li><li>Always wear your seat belt whenever you are in a car or truck</li><li>Avoid climbing ladders or going up on the roof</li><li>Hold handrails when you go up or down stairs</li><li>Never text while walking or driving</li></ul>
THE RISK:	After a head trauma, you lose your sense of smell
THE RESCUE:	Spend time sniffing essential oils, including rose, cloves, lemon, and eucalyptus, to help regain your sense of smell

SCARLETT SAYS: *If you've had a head trauma—a concussion or loss of consciousness, say—hyperbaric oxygen therapy might help. It involves spending time in a chamber where the air is up to double the normal pressure, which allows your body to absorb more healing oxygen.*

CONSIDER TAKING NUTRACEUTICALS

- ✓ A daily high-dose multivitamin/mineral complex with higher levels of vitamins B6, and B12, folate, and vitamin D
- ✓ Omega-3 fatty acids: 2.8 grams a day of total EPA plus DHA
- ✓ A daily combination of ginkgo biloba extract + acetyl-L-carnitine + huperzine A + N-acetylcysteine + alpha-lipoic acid + phosphatidylserine

EAT MORE OF THESE FOODS AND SPICES TO HEAL FROM HEAD TRAUMA

Spices and herbs to support brain healing, particularly turmeric and peppermint

Choline-rich foods to boost acetylcholine, such as shrimp, eggs, scallops, sardines, chicken, turkey, tuna, cod, beef, collard greens, and brussels sprouts

Omega-3-rich foods to support nerve cell membranes: See chapter 4

Other anti-inflammatory foods, such as prebiotic and probiotic rich foods: See chapter 4

Zinc-rich foods: See chapter 9

CHAPTER 6

RISK FACTOR: TOXINS

Exposure to environmental toxins has now been linked to health problems ranging from allergies and cancer to autoimmune and neurodegenerative diseases. That's because our bodies' systems to detoxify (through the gut, liver, kidneys, and skin), can become overwhelmed, damaging the brain, leading to serious illness and increasing the risk of memory problems and dementia.

YOUR PERSONAL RISK CHECKLIST:
Which Toxins Have You Been Exposed to?

Toxins can be absorbed through your skin, ingested (when you eat or drink), or inhaled. You may have been exposed to a toxin once, on occasion, or continuously. Below is a partial list of what you may have been exposed to. See chapter 10 in Memory Rescue for a more complete list.

- ☐ Tainted water
- ☐ BPA
- ☐ Heavy metals (such as lead, mercury from dental fillings, cadmium)
- ☐ Excessive alcohol
- ☐ Marijuana
- ☐ Medications (such as narcotics for pain, benzodiazepines for anxiety or insomnia)
- ☐ Chemotherapy
- ☐ General anesthesia
- ☐ Silicone breast implants that have leaked
- ☐ Artificial food dyes, preservatives, and sweeteners
- ☐ Herbicides
- ☐ Pesticides
- ☐ Health and beauty products (such as lead in lip products, formaldehyde in nail polishes)
- ☐ Air pollution
- ☐ Cigarette or marijuana smoke
- ☐ Vehicle exhaust
- ☐ Gasoline fumes

- ☐ Cleaning chemicals
- ☐ Welding or soldering fumes
- ☐ Fire retardant fumes
- ☐ Carbon monoxide
- ☐ Asbestos
- ☐ Fireplace fumes
- ☐ Paint and solvent fumes
- ☐ Pesticide and herbicide residues (farms, backyards)
- ☐ Mold

KEY TOXIN TESTS

The organs that detoxify your body—especially the liver, kidneys, and skin—need to be supported to do their job. The tests below will tell you how these organs are coping with your body's toxic load.

LIVER FUNCTION

- ☐ ALT (SGPT): Normal range: 7 to 56 units per liter (U/L)
- ☐ AST (SGOT): Normal range: 5 to 40 U/L
- ☐ Bilirubin: Normal range: 0.2 to 1.2 mg/dL
- ☐ Zinc: Normal range: 60 to 110 mcg/dL (low zinc will limit detoxification in the liver)

KIDNEY FUNCTION

- ☐ BUN: Normal range: 7 to 20 mg/dL
- ☐ Creatinine: Normal range: 0.5 to 1.2 mg/dL

SKIN

- ☐ Check for rashes, acne, and rosacea

TESTING FOR MOLD

- ☐ TGF beta-1: Normal level: below 2,380; 0 is optimal. Mold exposure can raise this to more than 15,000
- ☐ Real Time Labs mycotoxin test (http://www.realtimelab.com/home): for mold tests of human and environmental samples

HOW TO ADDRESS YOUR RISKS

THE RISK:	Exposure to toxins you ingest or absorb
THE RESCUE:	Try to limit your contact with toxins as much as possible: - Deal with drug abuse or alcohol dependence by examining the reasons you use - Gradually replace amalgam dental fillings with ceramic ones - Buy and eat organic foods as much as possible - Read and understand food labels to avoid additives like BHA, BHT, MSG, red dye #40, and artificial sweeteners - Buy food in glass, not plastic, containers - Limit alcohol to two to four servings a week - Eat more fiber: women: 21 grams a day; men: 30 grams daily - Drink 8 to 10 glasses of clean water daily - Do a food detox for 2 weeks
THE RISK:	Exposure to toxins you inhale
THE RESCUE	Try to limit your contact with toxins as much as possible: - Quit smoking (try hypnosis, nicotine patches) - Clean the air in your home: change filters on heating/cooling units, check for mold, avoid having wood fires in fireplace - Clean your home with fragrance-free natural household cleaners

THE RESCUE:	<ul><li>Avoid using products with volatile organic compounds (VOCs)—check air fresheners, paints, cleaning products and more</li><li>Replace aluminum and Teflon cookware (high heat may make Teflon release toxic fumes)</li></ul>

SCARLETT SAYS: *Toss out all your toxic beauty and health lotions and potions! Download the Think Dirty app (www.thinkdirtyapp.com) and scan your bathroom products to find out which ones are harmful.*

CONSIDER TAKING NUTRACEUTICALS

TO SUPPORT YOUR LIVER

- ✓ N-acetylcysteine (NAC)—600 mg twice a day
- ✓ Vitamin C: 1,000 mg twice a day
- ✓ Selenium: 200 micrograms (mcg) a day
- ✓ Zinc: 20 to 30 mg a day
- ✓ Folate (MTHF, methylfolate): 400 mcg a day
- ✓ Vitamin B12 (methyl cobalamin): 500 mcg a day
- ✓ Curcumin (in a bioavailable form like Longvida): 300 mg twice a day
- ✓ Artichoke extract

TO SUPPORT YOUR KIDNEYS

- ✓ Magnesium glycinate, citrate, or malate: 200 mg twice a day
- ✓ Curcumin: 300 mg twice a day
- ✓ Ginkgo biloba extract: 60 mg twice a day
- ✓ Fiber: seven grams (women) or ten grams (men) three times a day combined in food and supplements
- ✓ N-acetylcysteine (NAC): 600 mg twice a day
- ✓ Omega-3 fatty acids: 1.4 grams (or more) of a combination of EPA and DHA in about a 60/40 ratio

TO SUPPORT YOUR SKIN

- ✓ Vitamin D3: 2,000 IUs a day or more, depending on your level
- ✓ Vitamin E: 60 mg of mixed tocopherols a day
- ✓ Omega-3 fatty acids: 1.4 grams (or more) a day of a combination of EPA and DHA in about a 60/40 ratio
- ✓ CoQ10: 100 mg a day
- ✓ Alpha-lipoic acid: 300 to 600 mg a day
- ✓ Grapeseed extract: 100 to 300 mg a day
- ✓ EGCG: 600 mg a day
- ✓ Curcumin: 500 mg a day
- ✓ Selenium: 150 micrograms (mcg) a day
- ✓ Zinc: 25 mg a day
- ✓ Astaxanthin: 4 to 12 mg a day

SAM SAYS: *Get out and work up a sweat! It's one of your body's natural toxin-cleansing systems. Be sure to exercise and take saunas regularly.*

EAT MORE—OR LESS—OF THESE FOODS AND SPICES TO SUPPORT DETOXIFICATION

FOR A HEALTHIER LIVER

EAT MORE:

Green leafy vegetables (for folate)
Protein-rich foods, including eggs
Brassicas: any color cabbage, brussels sprouts, cauliflower, broccoli, kale for detox
Oranges and tangerines
Berries
Sunflower and sesame seeds
Caraway and dill seeds

EAT LESS:
Processed meats
Grapefruit
Capsaicin (from red chili peppers)
Conventionally raised produce
Dairy
Grain-fed meats
Farmed fish

FOR HEALTHIER KIDNEYS

EAT MORE:
Water
Spices to support detoxification: clove, rosemary, turmeric
Nuts and seeds: cashews, almonds, and pumpkin seeds for magnesium
Green leafy vegetables
Citrus fruits, except grapefruit
Beet juice
Ginger
Blueberries, raspberries, strawberries, blackberries
Garlic
Sugar-free chocolate

EAT LESS:
Too much animal protein
Excess salt
Excess phosphates (processed cheeses, canned fish, processed meats, flavored water, sodas, nondairy creamers, bottled coffee drinks and iced teas)

FOR HEALTHIER SKIN

EAT MORE:
Water
Green tea
Colorful fruits and vegetables for antioxidants: especially organic berries, kiwifruit, oranges, tangerines, pomegranates, broccoli, and peppers
Avocados
Olive oil
Almonds, walnuts, sunflower seeds
Wild salmon
Sugar-free chocolate

CHAPTER 7

RISK FACTOR: MENTAL HEALTH

The health of your mind is an essential factor in the health of your brain and memory. Mental health issues including depression, bipolar disorder, schizophrenia, attention deficit disorder/attention deficit hyperactivity disorder (ADD/ADHD), post-traumatic stress disorder (PTSD) and chronic stress can all contribute to a higher risk of memory, cardiovascular and other health problems. This is why you need to make sure your mind is as fit as it can be.

YOUR PERSONAL RISK CHECKLIST:
Which Mental Health Risk Factors Do You Have?

It is important to screen for mental health disorders to protect your brain and memory. One reason: When the elderly have depression, they may also show signs of cognitive impairment that can be misdiagnosed as dementia.

- ☐ ADHD
- ☐ Depression
- ☐ Bipolar disorder
- ☐ PTSD

KEY MENTAL HEALTH TESTS

See chapter 11 of Memory Rescue for the Amen Clinics' questionnaire concerning ADHD, depression, bipolar disorder, and PTSD. Depending on your score for each of these mental health problems, you may want to follow up with an evaluation by a psychiatrist or licensed counselor.

HOW TO ADDRESS YOUR RISKS

THE RISK:	Attention deficit hyperactivity disorder (ADHD)
THE RESCUE:	<ul><li>Adopt brain-healthy habits</li><li>Exercise</li><li>Try a higher-protein, lower-carbohydrate diet</li><li>Find an ADD/ADHD coach to work with</li><li>Take medication if you need it</li></ul>
THE RISK:	Depression
THE RESCUE	<ul><li>Adopt brain-healthy habits</li><li>Exercise</li><li>Eat a diet that is rich in antioxidants and tomatoes</li><li>Try cognitive behavioral therapy (CBT)</li><li>Get acupuncture</li><li>Take medication, if you need it (if you do, be sure to take methylfolate too)</li></ul>
THE RISK:	Bipolar disorder
THE RESCUE:	<ul><li>Adopt brain-healthy habits</li><li>Exercise</li><li>Take medication if you need it</li></ul>
THE RISK:	Post-traumatic stress disorder (PTSD)
THE RESCUE:	<ul><li>Adopt brain-healthy habits</li><li>Explore EMDR (eye movement desensitization and reprocessing; www.emdria.org)</li><li>Begin a loving-kindness meditation practice (see chapter 11 in Memory Rescue)</li><li>Take medication if you need it</li></ul>

THE RISK:	Too much stress
THE RESCUE:	<ul><li>Adopt brain-healthy habits</li><li>Exercise</li><li>Begin a prayer or mindfulness mecitation practice</li><li>When you wake up, say to yourself: "Today is going to be a great day"</li><li>Write down at least 3 things you feel grateful for every day</li><li>Walk in nature</li><li>Listen to soothing music</li><li>Keep a journal of your feelings</li><li>Drink green tea</li><li>Eat an ounce of dark chocolate</li><li>Turn off your mobile phone, tablet. and computer to reduce your daily screen time</li></ul>

SAM SAYS: *Make love with your spouse: It lowers stress hormones and may help your hippocampus, a key brain memory center (at least it does in mice!).*

CONSIDER TAKING NUTRACEUTICALS

FOR ADHD

- ✓ Omega-3 fatty acids (higher in EPA than DHA)
- ✓ Zinc
- ✓ Magnesium
- ✓ Iron (if ferritin levels are low)
- ✓ Phosphatidylserine

FOR DEPRESSION

- ✓ Omega-3 fatty acids (higher in EPA than DHA), especially when inflammation markers, such as CRP, are high
- ✓ SAMe (s-adenosyl methionine), especially in males
- ✓ Saffron
- ✓ Optimize vitamin D levels
- ✓ Magnesium

FOR BIPOLAR DISORDER

- ✓ Omega-3 fatty acids EPA and DHA

FOR STRESS

- ✓ Optimize your DHEA level to the high-normal range (see chapter 10)
- ✓ If you struggle with worry (the inability to let go of bothersome thoughts), consider supplements to raise the neurotransmitter serotonin, such as 5-hydroxytryptophan (5-HTP) or saffron
- ✓ If you struggle with anxiety (a pervasive sense of tension and nervousness), consider supplements to boost GABA, such as GABA itself, magnesium, and theanine from green tea

EAT MORE OF THESE FOODS AND SPICES TO HELP MENTAL HEALTH ISSUES

Spices to support mental health: saffron, turmeric (curcumin), saffron plus curcumin, peppermint (for attention problems), and cinnamon (for attention problems, ADHD, irritability)

Dopamine-rich foods for focus and motivation: turmeric, theanine from green tea, lentils, fish, lamb, chicken, turkey, beef, eggs, nuts, seeds (pumpkin and sesame), high-protein veggies (such as broccoli and spinach), and protein powders

Serotonin-rich foods for mood, sleep, pain, and craving control: Eat tryptophan-containing foods, such as eggs, turkey, seafood, chickpeas, nuts, and seeds (building blocks for serotonin) along with healthy carbohydrates, such as sweet potatoes and quinoa, to elicit a short-term insulin response that drives tryptophan into the brain. Dark chocolate also increases serotonin.

GABA-rich foods for anxiety: broccoli, almonds, walnuts, lentils, bananas, beef liver, brown rice, halibut, gluten-free whole oats, oranges, rice bran, and spinach

Choline-rich foods: See chapter 6

Fruits and vegetables for mood: Eat up to eight servings a day

Green tea

Maca: a root vegetable/medicinal plant, native to Peru, that has been shown to reduce depression

Omega-3-rich foods: See chapter 4

Antioxidant-rich foods: See chapter 3

Magnesium-rich foods for anxiety: See chapter 2

Zinc-rich foods: See chapter 9

Vitamin B6, B12, and folate-rich foods: See chapter 2

Prebiotic-rich foods: See chapter 4

Probiotic-rich foods: See chapter 4

CHAPTER 8

RISK FACTOR: IMMUNITY/INFECTION ISSUES

This risk factor is all about your body's defender, the immune system, which is always on the lookout for external invaders and internal troublemakers. When your immunity isn't what it should be, you may be more vulnerable to allergies, autoimmune disorders, and infections, and the last two can up your risk of brain fogginess ad memory issues.

YOUR PERSONAL RISK CHECKLIST:
Which Immunity and Infection Risk Factors Do You Have?

There are five types of immune system breakdowns, including immune deficiency disorders like HIV, allergies (to things like pet dander and peanuts), immune system cancers like lymphomas and leukemia, autoimmune disorders and infections. These last two, if left untreated, can cause serious memory problems and dementia.

- ☐ Autoimmune disorders such as multiple sclerosis, rheumatoid arthritis, systemic lupus erythematosus, Crohn's disease, psoriasis, Hashimoto's thyroiditis, and type 1 diabetes
- ☐ Infectious disease, including Lyme disease (and other tick-borne illnesses), toxoplasmosis, syphilis, Helicobacter pylori (H. pylori), HIV/AIDS, herpes

KEY TESTS OF IMMUNITY/INFECTIOUS DISEASE

- ☐ Complete blood count with differential
- ☐ Erythrocyte sedimentation rate (ESR
- ☐ Antinuclear antibodies (ANA)
- ☐ Rheumatoid factor (Rh
- ☐ Vitamin D: A normal level is 30 to 100 ng/mL; an optimal level is 50 to 100 ng/mL

☐ Screening for common infections: If your memory is not what it once was and you don't have the benefit of a SPECT scan, consider getting screened for infectious diseases that commonly affect memory, such as:
  - Borrelia burgdorferi (the spirochete that causes Lyme disease)
  - HIV/AIDS
  - Syphilis
  - Herpes simplex 1 and 2
  - Cytomegalovirus
  - Epstein-Barr virus
  - Toxoplasma gondii
  - Helicobacter pylori
  - Chlamydophila pneumoniae

HOW TO ADDRESS YOUR RISKS

THE RISK:	An infectious disease or autoimmune disease
THE RESCUE:	- Work with an integrative or functional medicine doctor who can properly diagnose and treat you - Try an elimination diet to see if food allergies are lowering your immunity (cut out sugar, gluten, dairy, corn, soy, additives, preservatives, artificial colors) - Consider getting tested for heavy metals - Address any gut issues you may have - Make sure your vitamin D levels are optimal - Manage your stress with laughter, among other strategies

CONSIDER TAKING NUTRACEUTICALS

✓ **Therapeutic mushrooms,** such as lion's mane, shiitake, reishi, and cordyceps
✓ **Aged garlic**
✓ **Anthocyanins:** fruit and vegetable extracts, blueberries, cranberries, grapes

- ✓ Echinacea
- ✓ Folate
- ✓ **Melatonin:** See chapter 12
- ✓ Probiotics
- ✓ Selenium
- ✓ Vitamin A
- ✓ Vitamin C
- ✓ Vitamin D3
- ✓ Vitamin E
- ✓ Zinc

EAT MORE OF THESE IMMUNITY-BOOSTING FOODS AND SPICES

Immunity-boosting spices: cinnamon, garlic, turmeric, thyme, ginger, coriander

Allicin-rich foods, including raw, crushed garlic, onions, and shallots

Quercetin-rich foods: red onions, red cabbage, red apples, cherries, red grapes, cherry tomatoes, teas, lemons, celery, and cocoa

Vitamin C–rich foods: natural blood thinners to boost circulation, including oranges, tangerines, kiwifruit, berries, red and yellow bell peppers, dark green leafy vegetables (such as spinach and kale), broccoli, tomatoes, peas

Vitamin D–rich foods: fatty fish, including salmon, sardines, tuna; eggs, beef liver, cod liver oil

Zinc-rich foods: oysters, beef, lamb, spinach, shiitake and cremini mushrooms, asparagus, sesame and pumpkin seeds

Mushrooms: shiitake, white button, portabella, morel, chanterelle

Selenium-rich foods: nuts (especially Brazil nuts), seeds, fish, grass-fed meats, mushrooms

Omega 3–rich foods: See chapter 4

Prebiotic-rich foods: See chapter 4

Probiotic-rich foods: See chapter 4

CHAPTER 9

RISK FACTOR: NEUROHORMONE DEFICIENCIES

Hormones are messengers—chemicals that are made by different parts of the body and sent to other areas to control your body's basic functions. The brain plays a significant role, both in sending out signals to release hormones and in being influenced by hormones from other areas of the body. Hormones work together in a delicate balance that can be upset if too much or too little of one or more is produced. You may experience symptoms that affect how you feel, think or act, and you may be more prone to depression, Alzheimer's disease, diabetes and other illnesses.

YOUR PERSONAL RISK CHECKLIST:
Which Neurohormone Risk Factors Do You Have?

There are literally hundreds of hormones that influence your brain, but these six are the most important: thyroid, cortisol, DHEA, estrogen, progesterone, and testosterone. Here are some of the risk factors you could have (you may not know you have one or more of them without laboratory testing):

- ☐ Underactive thyroid
- ☐ Overactive thyroid
- ☐ Elevated cortisol and Low DHEA (adrenal fatigue)
- ☐ Low estrogen
- ☐ Excess estrogen
- ☐ Low progesterone
- ☐ Perimenopause
- ☐ Menopause
- ☐ Low testosterone
- ☐ Excess testosterone

KEY NEUROHORMONE TESTS

For more detail on the following tests, see chapter 13 in Memory Rescue.

- ☐ Thyroid panel (includes TSH, Free T3, Free T4, and Thyroid antibodies)
- ☐ Liver function tests
- ☐ Ferritin level
- ☐ Cortisol
- ☐ DHEA-S (note that normal blood levels can differ by age and sex)
- ☐ Free and total serum testosterone (men and women)
- ☐ Estrogen and progesterone (women only)

SCARLETT SAYS: *To help avoid some of the problems that can arise with perimenopause, women should get their hormone levels checked at about age 35 to establish a baseline. From then on, get them rechecked every two to three years.*

HOW TO ADDRESS YOUR RISKS

THE RISK:	Hormones that are out of whack (too high or too low)
THE RESCUE:	Make it a priority to optimize your hormones by eliminating the things that harm them: • Quit smoking cigarettes if you are a smoker • Avoid processed food, excess sugar, wheat, and unhealthy fats • Cut back on caffeine and alcohol (limit: 2 to 4 servings a week) • Lose weight if you are overweight or obese Start engaging in healthier behaviors: • Exercise aerobically and lift weight • Get 7 to 8 hours of sleep every night • Try to manage your stress • Eat a healthy diet

THE RISK:	Exposure to endocrine disrupters, including BPA, phthalates, parabens and pesticides
THE RESCUE:	<ul><li>Buy organic food</li><li>Check the Environmental Working Group (www.ewg.org) for fruits and vegetables with the highest and lowest pesticide levels</li><li>Avoid buying and storing food in plastic containers</li><li>Limit or avoid conventionally raised produce and dairy</li><li>When taking hormone supplements, opt for bio-identical ones (they have fewer side effects)</li><li>See chapter 10 in Memory Rescue for additional suggestions</li></ul>

SAM SAYS: *Avoid drinking spearmint tea or eating soy and licorice as they all can lower your testosterone levels.*

CONSIDER TAKING NUTRACEUTICALS

For a more complete list of vitamins, minerals and herbal supplements for specific hormones, see chapter 11 in Memory Rescue.

- ✓ L-tyrosine: 500 mg two to three times a day
- ✓ Zinc: 20 to 30 mg a day
- ✓ DHEA: 10 mg a day or more (need determined by lab testing)
- ✓ Diindolylmethane (DIM): 75 to 300 mg a day
- ✓ Omega-3 fatty acids: 1,400 IU or more daily in a 60/40 ratio of EPA to DHA
- ✓ Calcium D-glucarate: 500 to 1,500 mg a day
- ✓ Probiotics: 3 billion live organisms a day, with both Lactobacillus and Bifidobacterium bacterial strains

EAT MORE OF THESE NEUROHORMONE-BALANCING FOODS AND SPICES

Fiber-rich foods, including those that contain lignin: green beans, peas, carrots, seeds, Brazil nuts

Hormone-supporting spices: garlic, sage, parsley, anise seed, red clover, hops

Eggs

Testosterone-boosting foods: pomegranates, olive oil, oysters, coconut, brassicas (including cabbage, broccoli, brussels sprouts, cauliflower), whey protein, garlic

Estrogen-boosting foods: soybeans, flaxseeds, sunflower seeds, beans, garlic, yams, foods rich in vitamins C and Bs, beets, parsley, aniseed, red clover, hops, sage

Thyroid-boosting (selenium-rich) foods: seaweed and sea vegetables, brassicas, maca

Progesterone-boosting foods: chasteberry, plus magnesium-rich foods (see chapter 2)

Zinc-rich foods to boost testosterone: See chapter 9

Prebiotic- and probiotic-rich foods: See chapter 4

CHAPTER 10

RISK FACTOR: DIABESITY

The word "diabesity" is combines diabetes and obesity, which are independent risk factors for failing memory and a number of forms of dementia. Diabetes damages blood vessels and eventually creates havoc throughout the body and brain, leading to Alzheimer's disease and vascular dementia, stroke, hypertension, and more. And overweight and obesity in midlife are associated with memory problems and dementia later in life. Obesity can contribute to diabetes risk, too.

YOUR PERSONAL RISK CHECKLIST:
Which Diabesity Risk Factors Do You Have?

- ☐ Aging
- ☐ Family history of diabetes
- ☐ Excessive consumption of sugar and high-glycemic foods
- ☐ Obesity
- ☐ Alcohol abuse
- ☐ Exposure to toxins
- ☐ Sedentary lifestyle
- ☐ Metabolic syndrome

KEY DIABESITY TESTS

- ☐ Body mass index (BMI): optimal is between 18.5 and 25; overweight is 25 to 30; obesity is over 30
- ☐ Waist to height ratio: calculate by dividing your waist size (in inches) by height (in inches); a healthy WtHR is under 50 percent
- ☐ Fasting blood sugar
    - •Normal: 70-105 mg/dL
    - •Optimal: 70-89 mg/dL
    - •Prediabetes: 105-125 mg/dL
    - •Diabetes: 126 mg/dL or higher

- ☐ Hemoglobin A1c (HBA1c)
  - •Normal: 4-5.6 percent
  - •Optimal: Under 5.3 percent
  - •Prediabetes: 5.7-6.4 percent
  - •Diabetes: Over 6.4 percent

- ☐ Fasting Insulin
  - •Normal: 2.6-25
  - •Optimal: Less than 10

SAM SAYS: *Get to know the glycemic index (GI), a helpful rating system that ranks carbohydrates on a scale of one to 100+ according to how they affect your blood sugar. Foods with a low ranking, like many vegetables, don't trigger blood sugar spikes, so they're better for you. Whenever possible, eat foods that have a GI under 60.*

HOW TO ADDRESS YOUR RISKS

THE RISK:	Being overweight and/or having a family history of diabetes
THE RESCUE:	<ul><li>Follow the Memory Rescue Diet</li><li>Limit low-fiber foods, sugar and foods that turn to sugar, wheat (and other grains), and processed foods</li><li>If you are overweight, lose weight slowly (one to two pounds a week)</li><li>Drink more water—and don't drink your calories</li><li>Take saunas to help detoxify</li><li>Exercise aerobically and lift weights</li><li>See your doctor to find out if medication is necessary</li></ul>

CONSIDER TAKING NUTRACEUTICALS

- ✓ **Omega-3 fatty acids:** 1.4 g (or more) daily of a combination of EPA and DHA in a 60/40 ratio
- ✓ **Chromium picolinate:** 200 to 1,000 micrograms (mcg) a day
- ✓ **Cinnamon:** 1 to 6 g a day as a supplement
- ✓ **Alpha-lipoic acid (ALA):** 300 to 600 mg a day
- ✓ **EGCG:** 500 to 800 mg a day (only take the higher dose under a doctor's supervision)
- ✓ **Magnesium:** 50 to 400 mg a day
- ✓ **Vitamin C**
- ✓ **Vitamin D**

EAT MORE OF THESE DIABESITY-FIGHTING FOODS AND SPICES

Spices: cinnamon, turmeric, ginger, cumin, garlic, cayenne, oregano, marjoram, sage, nutmeg

Fiber-rich foods to balance cholesterol and blood pressure: psyllium husk, navy beans, raspberries, broccoli, spinach, lentils, green peas, pears, winter squash, cabbage, green beans, avocados, coconut, fresh figs, artichokes, chickpeas, hemp seeds, and chia seeds

Polyphenol-rich foods/drinks, especially green tea, decaffeinated coffee, and blueberries. See chapter 8

Protein-rich foods: eggs, meats, fish

Vegetables: Best choices: celery, spinach, and brassicas (broccoli, brussels sprouts, cauliflower)

Fruits: apples, oranges, blueberries, raspberries, blackberries, and strawberries

Omega-3-rich foods: See chapter 4

Magnesium-rich foods: See chapter 2

Vitamin D–rich foods: See chapter 9

CHAPTER 11

RISK FACTOR: SLEEP ISSUES

Your brain needs sleep to stay healthy. New research has shown that during your slumbers your brain washes away waste and toxins that have accumulated during the course of the day. Chronic sleeplessness or insomnia raises your risk of everything from stroke to anxiety to cancer, and sleeping less than seven hours a night has been associated with a higher risk of dementia.

YOUR PERSONAL RISK CHECKLIST:
Which Sleep Risk Factors Do You Have?

- ☐ Insomnia
- ☐ Sleep apnea
- ☐ Poor sleep hygiene
- ☐ Shift work
- ☐ Depression
- ☐ Hormonal imbalances

KEY SLEEP TESTS

- ☐ Get evaluated for sleep apnea (If you snore loudly, stop breathing at night, or are chronically tired in the daytime)
- ☐ Assess the number of hours of sleep you need (find out how on chapter 15 of Memory Rescue)

HOW TO ADDRESS YOUR RISKS

THE RISK:	Health problems that can rob sleep
THE RESCUE:	Many conditions can disrupt sleep by making it harder to fall asleep, stay asleep, and more. If you have one of the following, discuss remedies with your health-care provider:

THE RESCUE:	- Sleep apnea - Restless leg syndrome - Thyroid conditions - Congestive heart failure - Chronic pain - Anxiety, depression and other untreated or undertreated mental health issues - Alzheimer's disease - Reflux and other gastrointestinal problems - Prostate problems
THE RISK:	Lifestyle habits that can lead to chronic insomnia Poor sleep hygiene
THE RESCUE:	- Cut out caffeine after 2 p.m. - Avoid nicotine, chocolate, and alcohol in the evening - Don't take daytime naps, which can further disrupt your sleep/wake cycle - Avoid eating a meal within two to three hours of going to bed - Finish vigorous exercise at least four hours before you head for bed
THE RISK:	Poor sleep hygiene
THE RESCUE:	- Make sure your bedroom is cool, dark, and quiet; use an eye mask or earplugs if you need them - Stash your gadgets (phone, tablets, digital watch) to block the screen light and sleep disruption

THE RESCUE:	<ul><li>Keep pets off the bed (and preferably out of the bedroom)</li><li>Go to bed at the same time and get up at the same time each night/day</li><li>Try to resolve emotional issues before going to bed</li><li>Establish a relaxing bedtime routine (warm bath or shower, warm almond milk, turn the lights low an hour beforehand)</li><li>Use your bed for sleep and sex—and nothing else</li><li>Avoid taking sleep meds like benzodiazepines</li></ul>

SCARLETT SAYS: *Scent your pillow case with lavender or keep a lavender pillow nearby. The aroma helps reduce anxiety and give you a better night's sleep.*

CONSIDER TAKING NUTRACEUTICALS

- ✓ **Melatonin:** 0.3–6 mg a day
- ✓ **5-HTP (especially for worriers):** 50–200 mg a day
- ✓ **Magnesium:** 50–400 mg a day
- ✓ **Zinc:** 20–40 mg a day
- ✓ **GABA:** 250–1,000 mg a day
- ✓ **Lemon balm (Melissa officinalis):** 300–600 mg a day
- ✓ **Vitamin D3:** 3,500 IU a day
- ✓ **Dr. Amen says:** My patients tend to like a combination of melatonin, magnesium, zinc, and GABA

EAT MORE OF THESE SLEEP-BOOSTING FOODS AND SPICES

Sleep-enhancing spices such as ginger root

Foods rich in melatonin (the hormone of sleep): tart cherry juice concentrate12 (also improves antioxidant status),13 cherries, walnuts, ginger root, asparagus

Serotonin-rich foods: See chapter 11

Magnesium-rich foods, which reduce anxiety. See chapter 2

Healthy carbohydrates, such as sweet potatoes, quinoa, and bananas (also high in magnesium)

Chamomile or passion fruit tea

PART III:
12 WEEKS TO A BETTER MEMORY

Finally! You are ready to start your personalized BRIGHT MINDS program. Just follow the steps here.

CHART YOUR BRIGHT MINDS RISK FACTORS

Fill out the chart below, using the information you have collected in chapters 1 through 11. Some sections will remain blank—for instance, if you are 45 years old, Retirement/Aging may not be a risk factor, or if you never hit your head or had a concussion, you would leave Head Trauma blank. Be sure to add the results of any additional testing you have had for your particular risk factors.

BRIGHT MINDS	MY RISK FACTORS	ADDITIONAL TEST RESULTS
Blood Flow		
Retirement/Aging		
Inflammation		
Genetics		
Head Trauma		

BRIGHT MINDS	MY RISK FACTORS	ADDITIONAL TEST RESULTS
Toxins		
Mental Health		
Immunity/Infection Issues		
Neurohormone Deficiencies		
Diabesity		
Sleep Issues		

DECIDE WHICH RISK FACTOR(S) TO TACKLE NOW

If you have more than one risk factor—that's not unusual!—it may feel daunting to take all of them on at once. Consider addressing the one that seems the most critical to you; see chapter 21 in Memory Rescue for further guidance on how to choose. As you progress on this 12-week program, you will address all of your personal risk factors and be able to look back at your accomplishments, knowing you have improved your brain, memory, and total health.

SUPPLEMENTS/NUTRACEUTICALS

Everyone should take basic, brain-healthy supplements daily, including:

- A 100% multivitamin/mineral complex plus extra vitamins B6 and B12, folate, and vitamin D
- Omega-3 fatty acids EPA and DHA

In addition, it's a good idea to take targeted nutraceuticals (supplements with medicinal properties). Studies have shown that high-quality, targeted nutraceuticals can have a positive impact on the brain. Check the lists of nutraceuticals for your risk factors to see which ones are recommended.

FOODS

- **Foods/Drinks to Add**
  In each of the previous BRIGHT MINDS risk factor chapters there is a list of recommended healthy foods. From the chapters that reflect your personal risk factors, select foods that you can begin to incorporate into your diet this week.

- **Foods/Drinks to Avoid or Eliminate: The Master List**
  Foods and beverages can be problematic for one or more of the BRIGHT MINDS risk factors, indicated by bold face highlighting in the list below. For example, alcohol should be limited or eliminated if any of the following risk factors pertain to you: Blood flow (B), Head trauma (H), Mental health (M), Immunity/Infections (I), or Sleep (S).

✓ Alcohol (**B**R**IGHT** **M**IND**S**)
✓ Aspartame (BRIGHT MINDS)
✓ Baked goods (BRIGHT MINDS)
✓ Black bean chili (BRIGHT MINDS)
✓ Caffeine (BRIGHT MINDS)
✓ Charred meats (BRIGHT MINDS)
✓ Corn, peas (BRIGHT MINDS)
✓ Dairy (BRIGHT MINDS)
✓ Dried fruits (BRIGHT MINDS)

- ✓ Excitotoxins, including MSG, aspartame, hydrolyzed vegetable rotein, sucralose, and "natural flavors" (BRIGHT MINDS) Energy drinks (BRIGHT MINDS)
- ✓ Food additives, such as MSG and aspartame (BRIGHT MINDS)
- ✓ Foods that contain diuretics, such as celery, cucumbers, radishes, and watermelon (BRIGHT MINDS)
- ✓ Foods that contain tyramine, such as tomatoes, eggplant, soy, red wine, and aged cheeses (BRIGHT MINDS)
- ✓ French fries and other fried foods (BRIGHT MINDS)
- ✓ Gluten (BRIGHT MINDS)
- ✓ Grain-fed meats (BRIGHT MINDS)
- ✓ Grapefruit (BRIGHT MINDS)
- ✓ High-glycemic, low-fiber foods (BRIGHT MINDS)
- ✓ High-glycemic fruits, such as pineapple, watermelon, and ripe bananas (BRIGHT MINDS)
- ✓ High omega-6 vegetables: corn and soybeans (BRIGHTMINDS)
- ✓ High omega-6 vegetables oils (BRIGHT MINDS)
- ✓ High protein foods because they're harder to digest (BRIGHT MINDS)
- ✓ Low-in-fiber fast foods (BRIGHT MINDS)
- ✓ Meals with high GI foods and lots of saturated fat (BRIGHT MINDS)
- ✓ Pesticide-laden foods (BRIGHT MINDS)
- ✓ Processed cheeses and microwave popcorn (BRIGHT MINDS)
- ✓ Processed foods (BRIGHT MINDS)
- ✓ Processed meats (BRIGHT MINDS)
- ✓ Protein from animals raised with hormones or antibiotics (BRIGHT MINDS)
- ✓ Refined grains (BRIGHT MINDS)
- ✓ Soda, regular and diet (BRIGHT MINDS)
- ✓ Soy protein isolate (BRIGHT MINDS)
- ✓ Spicy foods, especially at night (BRIGHT MINDS)
- ✓ Standard American diet (BRIGHT MINDS)
- ✓ Sugar and foods that turn to sugar (BRIGHT MINDS)
- ✓ Trans fats (BRIGHT MINDS)
- ✓ Unhealthy fatty foods, such as burgers, fries, and pizza, that have hard-to-digest saturated fats (BRIGHT MINDS)
- ✓ Wheat flour (BRIGHT MINDS)

EXERCISE

Everyone can benefit from at least 30 minutes of daily exercise. See chapter 2, for the specific kinds that have a payoff for your brain and whole body.

"RESCUE" INTERVENTIONS

Each risk factor chapter has a table of "Risks" and Rescues." Based on your risk factors, select the healthy actions you will take make your brain and your body healthier.

PART IV: RESOURCES

AMEN CLINICS:
www.amenclinics.com

BRAINMD:
To get more information on supplements go to www.brainmdhealth.com